SUMMARY

With ANALYSIS & ADDITIONS

SECRETS BEHIND CHRONIC and MYSTERY ILLNESS and HOW to FINALLY HEAL

MEDICAL MEDIUM

BY ANTHONY WILLIAM

SUMMARY BY:

ALTERNATE UNIVERSE BOOKS

Complete Chapter-by-Chapter Summary

ALTERNATE UNIVERSE
BOOKS

ISBN# 978-0-9726417-8-4

The author of this book does not diagnose, dispense or prescribe medical advice. Information herein is only offered in an anecdotal nature as part of your quest for improving emotional and spiritual well-being.

If you, or others, choose to use information from the contents of this book, the publisher assumes no responsibility for any and all consequences, direct or indirect.

You should always consult medical professionals before adopting any suggestions included in this book, or any conclusions you may draw from the contents.

This summary is meant to provide quick insight into the Medical Medium book. It also provides additional perspective.

Book Interior & E-book Formatting by Soumi Goswami |
soumi.goswami.pub@gmail.com

Dedicated to all those seeking truth in Spirituality, Health and Life…

CONTENTS

SUMMARY/ Anthony William INTRODUCTION

William asks…Do you need reassurance, are you seeking tools for prevention, have you tried everything, gone everywhere? This book contains these answers and you will not find them anywhere else.

The information comes from the heavens…from Spirit. Most of it has yet to be discovered. Included in this book is healing guidance that Spirit is revealing for the first time.

THE QUICKENING

Civilization is changing at a revolutionary pace, but also holds an era of danger. There are greater demands, pitfalls and responsibilities. Women bear the brunt, with chronic illness becoming a widespread issue.

There must be an interruption of the constant flow of information to help to stop unnecessary suffering. We must adapt by changing our health.

People stay sick because answers to the underlying issues of chronic illness and autoimmune disorders are not out there.

This book is a guide to the answers.

PUBLISHER'S INTRODUCTION

The intent of *Alternative Universe Books* is to bring to the reader a clear, accurate, and concise version of an original work. It is not an attempt to trash or demean the work of Anthony William and instead includes relevant additional information, where necessary.

There are Masters among us and it is with true discernment that we recognize them as such. The Masters are the checks and balances that guide the path of humanity. It is those checks and balances that keep us safe, and at times, healthy.

As a collective, *Alternative Universe Books*, possesses eons of knowledge in the areas of health and spirituality, and bring you unbiased information. This, in the hopes you will achieve your greatest desires from the words presented herein with analysis and additions where appropriate.

FOREWORD

BOOK SUMMARY/ KEY CONCEPTS

PART I WHERE IT ALL BEGINS ORIGINS OF THE MEDICAL MEDIUM

A 'Spirit' contacted Anthony William at a very young age. This Spirit whispered outside his right ear the health issues of those around him. This began with his Grandmother. The information was perplexing, and even difficult to endure at times. He attempts to resist the path the Spirit has offered him. Eventually, as a result of a near drowning for himself and his dog, he commits to do the work with the spirit in exchange for their lives. He is then taught to 'read' people's bodies and becomes the "Medical Medium."

William says he reveals health ideas and concepts not known to the medical community as yet.

KEY CONCEPTS PART II THE HIDDEN EPIDEMIC

- 'Mystery Illness'

The initial concept of the book covers something called 'Mystery Illness.' William lays out the three categories that these illnesses fall under as, *unnamed illnesses, ineffective treatment,* and *misdiagnosis.* All autoimmune disease falls under these categories and the book reveals his answers (or the Spirits') for healing them.

- Epstein-Barr Virus (EBV), the Hidden Epidemic

William writes that EBV is the underlying cause of most mystery illness. He describes the origins and transmission of the virus, as well as the four stages it goes through. The next chapters in this section include the illnesses that fall under the solved mystery.

- How to heal

Healing foods, supplements and herbs are listed as the answer.

PART III SECRETS BEHIND OTHER MYSTERY ILLNESSES

- Illnesses such as MS, RA, Hashimoto's, Diabetes and more, with descriptions as to how EBV is the underlying culprit. Additional lists of foods, supplements and herbs are given for healing each disorder.

PART IV HOW TO FINALLY HEAL

- The next chapters explain gut health and how to achieve it, detoxing the body, and what NOT to eat. Included is a chapter describing the 28-Day Healing-Cleanse.

- The next to the last chapter describes Soul-Healing Meditations and Techniques. These are various descriptions of every-day meditations to incorporate into your life.
- The final chapter closes with Essential Angels. The 'truth' about Angels; the twenty-one Essential Angels; and the Unknown Angels. The chapter finishes with how to access angelic aid.

CASE HISTORIES

At the end of each chapter of the original work is a case history. They consist of descriptions of the person's medical story and symptom picture, with few details to the specific treatment leading to the cure. For this reason, they have not been included.

PART I

WHERE IT ALL BEGINS

CHAPTER I

Origins of the Medical Medium

At four-years old, Anthony William has an encounter with a voice that says, *"I am Spirit of the Most High. There is no Spirit above me but God."*

The old man guides him with a beard in a brown robe (that no one else can see or hear) to put his hand on his Grandmother's chest. He is told to say, "Lung cancer." His Grandmother confirms weeks later, after a visit to the doctor, that she does in fact have lung cancer.

The voice comes to him every morning after that. Over time he is being told the health condition of everyone he encounters. When he resists the excess, disturbing information and inquires what this is really about, the Sprit explains he is a '*word*'. He says, "*The word is "Compassion", it is the closest word to God.*"

Words are an energy source, like Faith, Hope, Joy and Peace. Compassion is the closest word to God. These words need compassion to be complete because compassion is the understanding of suffering.

God is the word LOVE…which is above all other words. God loves all unconditionally.

He is told only one or two people per century are given this gift of communication with a Spirit. He will need to learn to become comfortable with the suffering of others, or chances are he will end his life, as others have in the past.

In time he is not only verbally told what is wrong with someone, but is helped to learn to see visual 'scans' of the persons' body.

As he matures, he gets a job in a grocery store, consults with people, and leads them to the foods and supplements in the store that they need to heal. In time he learns to read a person's emotional state first to see if they are approachable and can handle the information concerning their health.

Later Spirit teaches him how to identify herbs in nature and how to use them. Then he moves on to fixing cars, since there is no emotional attachment there. Spirit tells him how to find the issue and fix the cars.

He tries in many ways to get rid of Spirit, since this information is such a burden to him in his life. Finally, as a young man he accepts the hand he was dealt…that he has a special purpose and will accept it…for now.

Later, as he continues to be disgruntled, the final reckoning comes in the form of a near drowning. One day, as his dog jumps into the bay, he attempts to swim the frigid waters to save him. As the current is bringing them both down and he is pleading to Spirit for their lives, he is made to vow to succumb to his destiny. When Spirit, saves them both with the aid of an Angel, he commits to assume the role as the 'Medical Medium.'

His abilities increase after this and are now reading someone's soul, heart and spirit, besides their physical illness.

SOUL- consciousness of the person. Resides in the brain and stores memories, your hope and your faith. The soul can fracture, due to hardships.

HEART- where love, compassion and joy reside. Serves as your compass for your actions. Guides you when your soul becomes lost. Keeps a record of good intentions.

SPIRIT- your will and physical strength. Spirit can keep you physically going while you look for opportunities to heal.

CHAPTER II

The Truth About Mystery Illness

A mystery illness is any ailment that leaves you perplexed. This includes named diseases with no cure.

Autoimmune has become a 'mystery' disease. The body does not attack itself for any reason they just can't figure out the reason. Mystery illness is at an all-time high. Causes of symptoms often aren't evident.... no clear explanation. There are three categories:

Unnamed Illness- when the medical community can't figure out the source of your illness it becomes idiopathic, or worse yet, hypochondria.

Ineffective Treatment- a diagnosed illness with no avenue for recovery. There is no treatment, or no treatment that works on the person.

Misdiagnosis- when someone is given a named diagnosis, but it is flat out wrong. The treatment many times makes them worse.

FADS IN MEDICINE

Fads in medicine are Health trends that take hold until they prove to be incorrect. Examples, anti-biotics for Lyme disease; Hashimoto's being the immune system attacking itself; Candida being cured with a no-carb diet.

Knowing the cause of an illness is half the battle, how to make it better is the next step. Spirit has the answers.

PART II

THE HIDDEN EPIDEMIC

CHAPTER III

Epstein-Barr Virus, Chronic Fatigue Syndrome, and Fibromyalgia

A statistic is stated that out of 320 million people in the U.S., over 225 million have some form of Epstein-Barr Virus (EBV).

EBV is responsible for many mystery illnesses. The medical community is aware of one strain of EBV, however, there are over sixty varieties. These varieties of virus are responsible for fibromyalgia, chronic fatigue, thyroid disease, vertigo and other issues.

EBV ORIGINS AND TRANSMISSION

The virus was discovered and named in 1964, but was actually taking hold in the early 1900's. Initially it was only mildly harmful. Through the decades it has become more virulent.

Traditionally doctors have had no treatment until William brought to light answers for treatment.

HOW DO YOU CATCH EBV?

- Possibly from your mother as a baby if she was infected.

- Infected blood, since hospitals do not screen for this virus.
- Through a chef in a restaurant if he cuts a finger and is contaminated.
- Through bodily fluids from kissing or sex.

Transmission depends on the stage...EBV goes through four stages.

STAGE ONE

On transmission it goes through an initial dormant stage. It can become active if you are subjected to stress or stay dormant for days, months, or even years.

STAGE TWO

When activated, the virus turns into Mononucleosis. This is when it is most contagious. At this point the immune system goes to war tagging the invaders. The particular strain of EBV, or the strength of your immune system will determine the depth and length of your illness. During this stage the virus imbeds in an organ, such as the liver or spleen. The virus thrives on the toxins trapped in these organs.

EBV also has a relationship with the bacteria Streptococcus. When in the weakened state of contracting EBV the Strep can travel up to the throat and sinus or down to the urinary tract, vagina, kidneys or bladder.

STAGE THREE

Once the virus travels to an organ is settles there. Now a test shows antibodies from past infection, but misses the organ where it is lying dormant.

If you have an aggressive variety there can be serious problems, even while nesting. The organ it has invaded becomes inflamed.

The virus creates three types of poisons:

- Viral ***byproduct*** (poisons) that can show up as spirochetes. This can look like Lyme disease on screening tests.
- The ***corpse*** is the toxic dead cell at the end of its' six-week life cycle.
- ***Neurotoxins*** can be generated through the toxicity of the previous two. This can disrupt nerve function leading to more misdiagnosis.

Repercussions from an aggressive form of EBV:

- Sluggish liver
- Hepatitis C
- Lowered hydrochloric acid, creating a toxic intestinal tract, which results in bloating and constipation.
- Oversensitivity to foods

LUPUS

The immune system's response from EBV toxins triggers symptoms that become identified as falling into the Lupus category. Instead, it is the body's allergic reaction to the neurotoxins that elevate inflammatory markers.

HYPOTHYROIDISM and OTHER THYROID DISORDERS

The virus can and does travel. When it moves to the thyroid is creates many of the thyroid disorders, especially Hashimoto's and Graves'. The virus can burrow into the thyroid creating multiple symptoms and the virus is missed. It can however, be rejuvenated.

Thyroid nodules can be an attempt by the immune system to wall off the virus with calcium. Further disturbance can come in the form of cysts. If this occurs, it is important to eat calcium-rich foods, or the disturbance can lead to osteoporosis.

STAGE FOUR

The neurotoxins are excreted continuously at this point preventing your immune system from attacking the virus. If the virus leaves the thyroid it will inflame the central nervous system.

If there is severe emotional injury many other strange symptoms can appear, from heart palpitations to nerve pain. This stage causes massive confusion and is a major source of mystery illness. This is when the muscle, joint pain, tingling/numbness, back pain, migraines, fatigue and more show up.

Even female symptoms thought to be menopause can be triggered by stage four EBV.

CHRONIC FATIGUE SYNDROME

It is the Epstein-Barr virus. The neurotoxins from the virus inflame the central nervous system. The adrenals and digestive tract can also be attacked.

FIBROMYALGIA

The Epstein-Barr virus inflaming the central nervous system and nerves throughout the body cause these symptoms.

TINNITUS

William says tinnitus is Epstein-Barr virus getting into the ear nerve labyrinth.

VERTIGO and MENIERE'S DISEASE

The neurotoxins of the Epstein-Barr virus inflame the vegus nerve.

Two additional groups…

GROUP FIVE

Especially nasty and can develop as early as your twenties. Feeds on negative emotions.

GROUP SIX

Worst type, can even strike in young children. Can be misdiagnosed as leukemia, viral meningitis, Lupus and others. Symptoms include rashes, weak limbs, and severe nerve pain.

HEALING FROM EPSTEIN-BARR VIRUS

Healing period is three months to a year, sometimes eighteen months. Depends on your level of health.

HEALING FOODS

Eat three of these foods per day; rotate so that within a two-week period you've consumed all of them.

- Wild blueberries
- Celery
- Sprouts
- Asparagus
- Spinach
- Cilantro
- Parsley
- Coconut Oil
- Garlic
- Ginger
- Raspberries
- Lettuce
- Papayas
- Apricots
- Pomegranates
- Grapefruit

- Kale
- Sweet potatoes
- Cucumbers
- Fennel

HEALING HERBS and SUPPLEMENTS

- Cat's claw
- Silver hydrosol
- Zinc
- Vitamin B12
- Licorice root
- Lemon balm
- 5-MTHF
- Selenium
- Red marine algae
- L-lysine
- Spirulina
- Ester-C
- Nettle leaf
- Monolaurin
- Elderberry
- Red clover
- Star anise
- Curcumin

CHAPTER IV

Multiple Sclerosis

Starting in the 1950's mostly women were diagnosed with Multiple Sclerosis (MS). Once men began to be diagnosed, the medical community took notice.

MS is the name of a condition that inflames the myelin sheath, which protects the central nervous system.

There is no definitive test for diagnosing MS. Lesions in the brain or spinal cord is largely the evidence for doctors to conclude an MS diagnosis.

WHAT IS MS? A version of the Epstein-Barr virus! It is a virus attacking you and not your immune system.

- EBV inflames the nerves
- EBV is accompanied by fungi, bacteria and heavy metals

If you have MS, you will typically have EBV co-factors such as:

- Streptococcus
- H-pylori
- Candida
- Cytomegalovirus

- Heavy metals- copper, mercury and aluminum

The following supplements are recommended to reduce pain and protect the myelin sheath:

- EPA & DHA (Omega 3 Fats)
- L-glutamine
- Lion's mane
- Alpha lipoic acid
- Monolaurin
- Curcumin
- Barley grass juice extract powder

William states that if you stick to the recommendations you can restore your central nervous system typically in 3-18 months. Time frame is based on your current state of health.

CHAPTER V

Rheumatoid Arthritis

Rheumatoid arthritis or RA affects the small joints in the hands, feet, knees, elbows and other larger joints. It can also affect nerves, skin, eyes, mouth, lungs and heart. The affliction results in joint pain and swelling. Joint deformity may occur.

RA is another 'dis-ease' that falls under the category of auto-immune. It is believed to be an attack by the immune system on itself, however; the inflammation is there to protect the joints from a common virus.

Tests commonly used to identify RA:

- Rheumatoid factor blood test
- Anti-cyclic citrullinated peptides- antibody blood test
- Erythrocyte sedimentation rate blood test
- C-reactive protein blood test
- Ultrasounds
- MRI's

None are reliable, since they miss any evidence of virus.

WHAT RA REALLY IS?

The medical community believes it to be the body attacking itself. It is however, a form of Epstein-Barr virus.

HEALING FROM RA

The typical medications comprised of painkillers and steroids do not address the underlying cause. Prescription drugs actually lower the immune system, hindering it further from fighting the virus.

The following are natural anti-inflammatory to help alleviate pain and promote healing (along with the use of the supplements listed in Chapter III.)

- Curcumin
- Nettle leaf
- Turmeric
- N-acetyl cysteine
- MSM

Also use cold and hot packs (cold for 30 minutes, hot for 10 minutes.) Add to this the protocol listed in Part IV. The time frame listed is a few months to two years for recovery.

CHAPTER VI

Hypothyroidism and Hashimoto's Thyroiditis

Thyroid disease, specifically goiters, did not appear until the beginning of the industrial revolution at the turn of the 19th Century. They are a result of nutritional deficiencies such as zinc, iodine or from heavy metals. The increase in toxicity created more cases of goiters.

At the turn of the 20th century the food supply began to be stripped of nutrients and packed in lead-lined cans. Lead also produced goiters.

Fast-forward to the use of dried thyroid gland from pigs as medicine to relieve the thyroid disorders. This helped to replenish necessary iodine and created the first steroid compound to suppress inflammation (and the immune system).

In the 20th century women showed up to a different thyroid disorder, now named *thyroiditis* (inflamed thyroid). Today it is referred to as Hashimoto's or hyperthyroidism. They are part of the mystery illness category.

UNDERSTANDING HYPOTHYROIDISM AND HASHIMOTO'S

The thyroid is a tiny very important gland in the neck. It regulates how much or how little energy you take in. This affects every cell in the body.

When the thyroid operates smoothly, so do you, if not, health issues arise. Hypothyroidism is the name attached to underproduction of hormones. This condition, along with Hashimoto's, is the condition that brought on goiters in years gone by. The new names do not explain the fatigue, palpitations, hot flashes, brain fog, weight gain and other symptoms associated with them.

Ninety-five percent of today's thyroid disorders are from the viral infection Epstein-Barr. Sometimes after a long incubation period in the liver the virus moves to the thyroid. It will then inflame the thyroid and symptoms will go from hypothyroidism to the diagnosis of Hashimoto's. The immune system is actually going after an intruder, the virus, hence the change in symptoms.

Thyroid medications do not go after the root-cause; they just add hormones to the bloodstream. This is in the hopes they will replace the hormones the thyroid is not producing.

Medication can give relief and act as a Band-Aid, but when symptoms do not improve it is the virus that needs treating.

Follow the program in Chapter III to get rid of the Epstein-Barr virus. The advice below can help to heal and protect your damaged thyroid and fortify supporting glands.

THYROID BLOOD TESTS

- TSH,
- Free T4,

- Free T3
- Thyroid antibodies

If thyroid tests reveal normal range, there can still be an issue. Regardless of test results, there can still be low-grade viral symptoms not picked up for years. If you have thyroid symptoms, regardless of lab tests, use the programs in Chapter IV and Part IV, as well as the next section.

ADDRESSING THYROID CONDITIONS

Foods, herbs and supplements can heal your damaged thyroid and strengthen your endocrine system.

"Goitrogenic Foods"

A new fad idea about cruciferous vegetables is discouraging people from eating cauliflower, kale, broccoli, cabbage and other foods that contain goitrogens. You'd have to eat barrels full to be affected so disregard this latest trend.

HEALING FOODS

The following work to kill EBV cells; provide micronutrients, repair thyroid tissue, reduce nodule growth, flush heavy metals and viral waste and boost production of thyroid hormones.

- Atlantic dulse
- Wild blueberries
- Sprouts
- Cilantro
- Garlic
- Hemp seeds
- Coconut oil

- Brazil nuts
- Cranberries

HEALING HERBS AND SUPPLEMENTS

- Zinc
- Spirulina
- Bladderwrack
- Chromium
- L-tyrosine
- Ashwagandha
- Licorice root
- Eleuthero (Siberian Ginseng)
- Lemon Balm
- Manganese
- Selenium
- Vitamin D3
- B-Complex
- Magnesium
- EPA & DHA
- Bacopa monnieri
- Rubidium
- Copper

PART III

SECRETS BEHIND OTHER MYSTERY ILLNESSES

CHAPTER VII

Type II Diabetes and Hypoglycemia

Glucose is the fundamental fuel our body runs on. It is a simple sugar that provides energy to every cell in order to function. Cells don't access glucose directly, but employs the help of the pancreas. The pancreas monitors your blood and produces insulin as needed. Extra glucose is stored in the liver. If you have a strong liver, it is released for use by your cells.

If the pancreas fails to produce enough insulin and/or cells refuse to let in glucose from the blood, insulin resistance sets in. Some of the excess glucose in the blood can be expelled through frequent urination. You can also begin to get thirsty from dehydration. These issues can set you up for Type II diabetes.

WHAT REALLY CAUSES TYPE II DIABETES AND HYPOGLYCEMIA

Excess adrenaline causes damage to the pancreas. The pancreas can then no longer produce enough insulin to remove glucose from the blood. The adrenaline/insulin blend causes a disruption, which leads to lowered insulin production and non-acceptance of glucose in the cells.

If adrenals produce too little adrenaline, the pancreas works overtime to compensate. The pancreas becomes inflamed trying to compensate, one-way or the other. The pancreas also is responsible for digestive enzymes, which are now in danger and can create digestive issues.

Hypoglycemia can be the precursor to type II diabetes as the glucose levels begin to fluctuate abnormally. The food choices you make also contribute. Fat can strain the liver and pancreas more than sugar consumption. There will be insulin resistance from high levels of blood fat after a high protein-fat meal that stops the body's ability to allow insulin produced by the pancreas to drive sugar into the cells. Now there is too much sugar in the blood with the liver having to try to store it. If the liver dumps it back into the blood hypoglycemia occurs.

ADDRESSING TYPE II DIABETES AND HYPOGLYCEMIA

Animal fats weaken the pancreas and liver, while sugar was the messenger. To address type II diabetes and hypoglycemia it is important to lower animal fat consumption and instead raise fresh fruit and vegetable intake.

The cleanse in Chapter XXII will help to heal the liver, pancreas, and adrenal glands in stabilizing blood sugar levels. When insulin is given it lowers blood glucose level, but does not address the main issue of damage to the adrenals and damaged pancreas, dysfunctional liver, insulin resistance and even chronic negative emotions.

BOLSTER YOUR ADRENAL GLANDS

The length of the program is determined by the amount of damage needing attention. Check out Part IV also, for added guidance. Read Chapter IX, "Adrenal Fatigue" to work on any adrenal damage.

HEALING FOODS

How to detox the liver, strengthen glucose levels, support the pancreas, boost adrenals, and stabilize insulin. Avoid cheese, milk, cream, butter, eggs, processed oils and all sugars (except raw honey and fruit).

Top foods for type II diabetes:

- Wild blueberries
- Spinach
- Celery
- Papayas
- Sprouts
- Kale
- Asparagus

HEALING HERBS AND SUPPLEMENTS

- Zinc
- Chromium
- Spirulina
- Ester-C
- Alpha lipoic acid
- Silica
- Purslane
- Eleuthero (Siberian Ginseng)
- Panax ginseng
- EPA & DHA
- Biotin
- B-Complex
- Gymnema sylvestre
- Magnesium
- Vitamin D3

CHAPTER VIII

Adrenal Fatigue

The adrenal glands sit on top of the kidneys. They are responsible for producing adrenaline, cortisol, and hormones, such as estrogen and testosterone. Adrenals can become damaged as a result of too much stress, which creates excess adrenaline. At this point they react erratically.

Fatigued adrenals can affect the heart, pancreas, liver and central nervous system. Hypothyroid symptoms, such as weight gain, depression, hair loss, brittle nails, etc. can occur when there is also too little cortisol.

AVOIDING ADRENAL FATIGUE

- Avoid excess stress
- Avoid artificial stimulants
- Avoid painful emotions, embrace joyful ones

ADDRESSING ADRENAL FATIGUE

Recovering can take from one month to two and a half years depending on the extent of damage. Access suggestions in Part IV also.

EXTERNAL CORTISOL: FOR EMERGENCIES ONLY

If you are in a state of crisis, a quick fix that may be recommended by your doctor is cortisol replacement medicine. Ultimately it is an immunosuppressant that weakens your immune system.

GRAZE EVERY ONE AND A HALF TO TWO HOURS

Eat light, balanced meals every ninety-minutes to two hours. Frequent meals keep your blood sugars up so adrenals don't have to interfere.

Snacks between meals should contain potassium, sodium, and natural sugars.

- A date, two celery sticks, an apple
- Half an avocado, spinach and an orange
- A sweet potato, parsley and lemon squeezed on kale

HEALING FOODS

- Sprouts
- Asparagus
- Wild blueberries
- Bananas
- Garlic
- Broccoli
- Kale
- Raspberries
- Blackberries
- Romaine lettuce
- Red-skinned apples

WHAT NOT TO EAT

High amounts of fat strain your pancreas and liver.

HEALING HERBS AND SUPPLEMENTS

- Licorice root
- Spirulina
- Ester C
- Chromium
- Eleuthero (Siberian Ginseng)
- Schisandra
- Ashwagandha
- Magnesium
- 5-MTHF
- Cordyceps
- Panax ginseng
- Rose hips
- Barley grass juice extract powder
- Astragalus
- Lemon balm
- Rhodiola

CHAPTER IX

Candida

William discusses the inaccurate diagnosis of Candida as an illness. That we all, in fact, have Candida and it is a natural, healthy fungus. Candida is a cofactor of Lyme, Shingles, EBV, Herpes, c.difficile, Streptococcus, H-pylori, Diabetes, MS, HHV-6, Cytomeglia virus and more.

Candida can be an indicator that there is something wrong, but is not the problem itself. Candida has become a convenient scapegoat.

THE TRUTH ABOUT CANDIDA

Candida causes very little harm and very few cases need treating. *(NOT TRUE- Candida destroys the myelin sheath)*

CANDIDA AND LEAKY GUT SYNDROME

William does not believe it to be true that Candida cuts through the lining of the intestines and colon resulting in leaky gut. He instead states the worse Candida can do is cause calluses on irritated portions of the intestinal tract. He believes this is as bad as it gets. Other issues are missed when there is focus on Candida.

FEAR OF FRUIT

Fruit binds with compounds like antioxidants that kill off Candida. Fruit sugar leaves the stomach in three to six minutes and does not touch the intestinal tract. The pulp, fiber, skin and seeds kill yeast.

Publisher's Note: *If this were true you would be devoid of circulation. See further notes in 'Conclusion'.*

THE FAT AND PROTEIN MYTH

William states that a high-fat, high-protein diet does not starve Candida, but feeds it. Proteins are inflammatory as is the issue of undigested proteins. The best anti-Candida approach is a low-fat, low-protein diet with plenty of fruits and vegetables.

HEALING FROM CANDIDA

If you are certain you have no other health issue other than Candida, follow the advice in Chapter XVIII "Gut Health." Increase hydrochloric acid, rebuild the intestinal tract and strengthen and detoxify the liver. Avoid antibiotics and antifungal medications.

CHAPTER X

Migraines

MIGRAINE TRIGGERS

Many times there are a combination of triggers.

- Concussion
- Meningitis
- Stroke
- Transient ischemic attack
- Brain aneurysm
- Brain Tumor
- Brain cyst
- Impeded cervical nerves
- Electrolyte deficiency
- Stress
- Hormone imbalance
- Sleep disorders
- Heavy metals

William states Epstein-Barr and Shingles are the main triggers. EBV can inflame the nervous system and Shingles can inflame your trigeminal and/or phrenic nerves. See Chapter IV for EBV symptoms and Chapter XII for Shingles symptoms.

FOOD TRIGGERS

- Eggs
- Dairy
- Gluten
- Meat

- Fermented foods
- Salt
- Oils
- Additives
- Alcohol
- Chocolate

ADDRESSING MIGRAINES

The most helpful thing is to eliminate triggers. Herbs and supplements, as well as healing foods can help to eliminate triggers. They can help to lower pain and inflammation, detox, soothe nerves, and improve gut health.

HEALING FOODS

Top foods for addressing migraines:

- Fresh celery juice
- Cilantro
- Hemp seeds
- Papayas
- Chili peppers
- Garlic
- Ginger
- Kale
- Cinnamon
- Apples

HEALING HERBS AND SUPPLEMENTS

- Chrysanthemum tea
- Fever few
- Butterbur
- Magnesium
- Ester C
- Ginkgo biloba
- White willow bark
- Kava-kava
- Lemon balm
- Rosemary leaf
- Riboflavin (Vitamin B2)
- Co-Enzyme Q10
- Cayenne pepper
- Skullcap
- Valerian root

CHAPTER XI

Shingles, True Cause of Colitis, TMJ, Diabetic Neuropathy, and More

Varieties of Shingles are responsible for Bell's palsy, frozen shoulder, diabetic nerve pain, colitis, vaginal burning, TMJ, Lyme disease, and misdiagnosed MS. There are actually thirty-one varieties. There are eight strains that produce NO rash.

TRANSMISSION & TRIGGERS

William states that, contrary to medical science, chicken pox has no connection to the Shingles virus, even though they are both in the Herpes family. The virus can lay dormant in your system for as long as 10-50 years. It typically hides in the liver until the immune system is triggered and it can rise up. This can be from a physical or emotional trigger.

SHINGLES WITH RASHES

Seven strains cause rashes and usually the location determines which one. It can attack on the upper body, arms, head, legs and even vaginal area. This last one is usually mistaken for Herpes. The neurotoxin of the virus causes the rashes, pustules and discomfort. There can be nerve damage, but most can drive it out.

SHINGLES WITHOUT RASHES

Eight strains do not cause rashes. In these cases, the neurotoxin does not come outward, but instead travels inward. There is a greater strain on the immune system. Immuno-suppressants and steroids can make these strains much worse. Antibiotics can be a double-blow to the immune system.

OTHER FORMS OF SHINGLES VIRUS

- Diabetic neuropathy- there is no link to diabetes. (Both nerve related issues).
- Maddening itch Shingles- a moving itch that can't be scratched, it is internal.
- Vaginal Shingles- goes deep and inflames the nerves.
- Colitis Shingles- steroids will only put it in remission.
- Arm & leg burning Shingles- nerve inflammation far below the skin.
- Mouth Shingles, TMJ, Bell's palsy- the virus affects the gums.
- Frozen shoulder Shingles- virus aggravates the nerves in the shoulder.
- Body on fire Shingles- every part of the body feels like it is on fire.

HEALING FOODS

Eat well, exercise and eat these healing foods daily.

- Wild blueberries
- Coconuts
- Papayas
- Red-skinned apples
- Pears
- Artichoke
- Bananas
- Sweet potato
- Spinach
- Asparagus
- Lettuce (deep green or red)
- Green beans
- Avocado

HEALING HERBS AND SUPPLEMENTS

- Alpha lipoic acid
- Magnesium
- MSM
- Vitamin B12
- EPA & DHA
- Lobelia
- Feverfew
- California poppy
- Licorice root
- Zinc
- L-lysine
- Selenium
- Nettle leaf

CHAPTER XII

Attention-Deficit/ Hyperactivity Disorder and Autism

A mother's intuition is the best tool for identifying these issues.

HIDDEN UPSIDES OF ADHD & AUTISM

Girls will more often have inattentiveness and ADD gets missed because they are categorized as 'ditzy' or 'spacey.' Hyperactivity is more often reserved for boys in the form of ADHD. Kids can shift between both of these disorders.

These children usually have a high level of intuition, creativity and the skill to 'read' people at a deeper level. They will grow up better equipped to solve humanities' problems.

CAUSES OF ADHD & AUTISM

Toxic heavy metals...mercury and aluminum that settles in the brain's midline cerebral canal. This divides the two hemispheres. (Mercury is also responsible for seizure disorders.)

Mercury can be transmitted from the mother while in the womb and from fathers at conception.

Cerebral Midline Canal

A channel of energy runs through this canal. It has not yet been discovered that the energy sets up communication between the hemispheres. It is how children see angels and imaginary friends. Heavy metals block the electrical and metaphysical transmissions. These interruptions cause neurons to fire that should not fire until after the age of eighteen.

Autism is a more advanced form of ADHD. The accumulation of heavy metals in this area of the brain determines the severity of the disorder. The extra materials block internal communication and the 'odd' behavior is the child learning to access different parts of themselves.

Specially Evolved Brain Neurons

These children grow specially evolved brain neurons, especially in the frontal lobe. As a result, they possess intuitive abilities. The neurons also evolve in the limbic system, altering behaviors, emotions and desires.

Age and Brain Development

The situation created by the heavy metals sets up by age four and can be removed if dealt with before the age of eighteen. By this age, the midline closes limiting the free-flow of energy. This is part of the maturing process, however, the metals become trapped.

PUBLISHER'S NOTE: The mid-line NEVER closes, if it did the left and right side of the brain would no longer communicate.

If you are an adult dealing with ADD, ADHD, or autism that interferes with your life, you can follow the advice in the next section to lessen its effects.

Addressing ADHD & Autism

Amphetamines are the conventional method of treating these conditions. Children are calmed for short periods of time. Most of these children do not get enough glucose to the brain. Amphetamines stimulate the adrenal glands to stimulate adrenaline, which the brain uses in place of glucose. The adrenaline forces electrical nerve impulses to fire at a much higher rate, stabilizing the child temporarily.

Unfortunately, the amphetamines place a heavy burden on the adrenals and other organs, causing them to be unstable over time. Ample fresh organic fruit is a better choice. If you remove grains and sugars from the diet, be sure to replace them with fruits. The high-fat ketogenic diet is also not a good choice and the results will be temporary.

The daily diet should consist of herbs, supplements and the foods that follow.

HEALING FOODS

The following is a food list to help flush heavy metals and other toxins, while supporting normal neuron transmission.

- Wild blueberries
- Cilantro
- Coconut oil
- Celery
- Bananas
- Blackberries
- Avocados
- Strawberries
- Flax seeds

HEALING HERBS AND SUPPLEMENTS

- Spirulina
- Vitamin B12
- Ester-C
- Zinc
- Melatonin
- Lemon Balm
- Magnesium
- Ginkgo biloba
- GABA
- B-Complex
- Ginseng
- Probiotics
- EPA & DHA

CHAPTER XIII

Posttraumatic Stress Disorder

UNRECOGNIZED PTSD

PTSD negatively influences our choices, no matter the scale of the incident. It changes who we are. Illness can create this issue, just as easily as other situations. With the right nutritional, emotional and soul-healing support, you can reclaim your operating capacity.

WHAT REALLY HAPPENS

A chemical imbalance in the brain occurs when there is trauma. If there is not enough *glucose* stored in brain cells to feed the nervous system, there can be lasting effects. It is glucose, rather than a loss of electrolytes, that is the cause. Glucose places a protective coating over sensitive neurological tissue.

- Glucose is needed to prevent the acidic nature of adrenaline and cortisol from saturating brain tissue.
- Glucose stops the electrical storm that arises from trauma with exaggerated electrical impulses.

HEALING PTSD

Lingering negative feelings that remain after an adverse incident can limit a person in many ways. Creating new, positive experiences can help to unburden the trauma. The more you create, the more you re-seed the brain. They don't have to be big; it is how you perceive them that retrain the brain.

Healing PTSD requires loving support, time, patience and nutritional elements. Part IV, 'How to Finally Heal,' imparts more on the subject. Prayer can also be your Angel of Restitution. The soul-healing meditations in Chapter XXIII can be of help.

HEALING FOODS

To restore glucose to the brain:

- Wild blueberries
- Melons
- Beets
- Bananas
- Persimmons
- Papayas
- Sweet potatoes
- Figs
- Oranges
- Mangoes
- Tangerines
- Apples
- Raw honey
- Dates

HEALING HERBS AND SUPPLEMENTS

- 5-MTHF
- B-complex
- Ginkgo biloba
- GABA
- Spirulina
- Honeysuckle
- Nettle leaf
- Siberian ginseng
- L-glutamine

CHAPTER XIV

Depression

DEPRESSION SYMPTOMS

- Sadness
- Loss of interest in activities
- Slow thinking, speaking or movement
- Thoughts of self-harm

IDENTIFYING AND ADDRESSING MAJOR CAUSES OF DEPRESSION

Many causes, emotional and/or physical

- Traumatic loss
- Traumatic stress
- Adrenal dysfunction
- Viral infection
- Heavy metals
- Non-metal toxins
- Electrolyte deficiency

HEALING FROM DEPRESSION

Start by addressing any known cause. Take the herbs, foods and supplements described in this section. Utilize the meditation techniques and exercises in Chapters XXIII & XXIV.

HEALING FOODS

- Wild blueberries
- Hemp seeds
- Cilantro
- Walnuts
- Coconut oil
- Sprouts
- Kale
- Apricots
- Avocados

HEALING HERBS & SUPPLEMENTS

- Vitamin B12
- Spirulina
- Nascent iodine
- Melatonin
- Ester-C
- Licorice root
- Ginkgo leaf
- Lemon balm
- Ashwagandha
- Vitamin D3
- GABA
- EPA & DHA
- 5-HTP
- B-complex
- Magnesium
- California poppy
- Kava-kava
- Vitamin E
- Rhodiola

CHAPTER XV

Premenstrual Syndrome and Menopause

William states that a woman's aging process is from puberty to menopause and actually slows down after menopause.

PUBLISHER'S NOTE: *We believe William has confused development with aging.*

He further states that by reducing hormone levels women are safeguarded against cancers, virus, and bacteria, which all feed on reproductive hormones.

PUBLISHER'S NOTE: *This scenario would only occur in an unhealthy state.*

Osteoporosis develops over decades and shows itself at menopause. He states that lowered levels of estrogen actually help bone density, since hormones are steroids and have a bone-dissolving affect.

PUBLISHER'S NOTE: *If this were the case all women would suffer from osteoporosis.*

Combined infections such as Epstein-Barr, nutritional deficiencies, inadequate exercise, estrogen, and progesterone can trigger osteoporosis long before menopause. It just happens to show up after menopause. Menopause is the body's natural way of slowing down aging.

WHAT'S REALLY BEHIND MENOPAUSE SYMPTOMS

- William states that women did not show symptoms of menopause until the 1950's. They were born at the time Epstein-Barr began to take root in the population.
- Radiation exposure was rampant in the 1950's due to the fluoroscope.
- X-ray boxes at the shoe stores from the 1920's – 1950's!
- DDT exposure, which began in the 1940's.

Menopause, and lowered hormones, became the scapegoat for the new symptoms not previously seen in other generations.

THE TRUTH ABOUT HORMONE REPLACEMENT THERAPY

HRT produces results by acting as a steroid, suppressing the immune system's response to viral inflammation, nutritional deficiencies, and exposure to toxins. In other words, it helps to hide disease.

The 2002 study, Women's Health Initiative, concluded that HRT substantially increased the risk of breast cancer, heart attacks, and strokes. Unfortunately, these results brought into being Bio-identical Hormone Replacement Therapy instead!

Saliva, blood and urine are not reliable tests for measuring hormone levels and can be grossly inaccurate. If the thyroid is out of balance, as well as adrenals, the accuracy of the results is skewed.

UNDERSTANDING MENOPAUSE TODAY

Younger women, at alarming rates, are experiencing hormonal and/ or peri-menopause symptoms. They are the same symptoms of Epstein-Barr, thyroid dysfunction, and toxic exposures. These underlying factors also interfere with achieving accurate results on hormone tests.

PUBLISHER'S NOTE: *This may also be due to previous pharmaceutical drug interventions.*

UNDERSTANDING PREMENSTRUAL SYMPTOMS

Depression, diarrhea, bloating, anxiety, insomnia, migraines and mood swings are not necessarily part of PMS. They are instead, the result of underlying health conditions. William says they are instead a sensitive central nervous system, IBS, food allergies, or heavy metal poisoning. The symptoms show up during menstruation because the immune system is overburdened and cannot keep them at bay.

To address symptoms associated with PMS, Menopause and Post-menopause:

HEALING FOODS

- Wild blueberries
- Sesame tahini
- Avocado
- Black beans
- Asparagus
- Apples
- Spinach
- Black grapes
- Cucumbers

HERBS AND SUPPLEMENT TO ADDRESS GENERAL SYMPTOMS

- Silver hydrosol
- Zinc
- Licorice root
- L-lysine
- Vitamin B12
- Nascent iodine
- Ashwagandha
- Barley grass juice powder
- Olive leaf
- Monolaurin
- Spirulina
- Ginseng

HERBS AND SUPPLEMENTS FOR THE REPRODUCTIVE SYSTEM

- Nettle leaf
- Wild Yam (raises estrogen)
- Schisandra berry
- Hawthorn berry
- Vitex (chaste tree berry)
- Red clover blossom
- Sage
- Folic acid
- B-complex
- Vitamin D3
- Vitamin E
- EPA & DHA

CHAPTER XVI

Lyme Disease

WHAT LYME DISEASE REALLY IS

Originally Lyme was attributed to a bacteria carried by deer, *Borrelia burgdorferi.* Recently focus has moved to a different bacterium, *Bartonella* and the microscopic parasite *Babesia.* William states these are all harmless, and we all carry them. The latter two have never been found in a tick.

William states it is actually viral! Each person affected has a different variation. Some have Epstein-Barr, some have HHV-6, others have different strains of Shingles, or Cytomegalovirus, etc. They all cause similar symptoms and are all in the Herpes family.

Any number of things can trigger the symptoms to develop… heavy metal toxicity, stress, or anything else that attacks the immune system. Your over-all health plays a role in how much you are affected or not affected by exposures.

COMMON LYME TRIGGERS

- MOLD
- MERCURY-BASED DENTAL AMALGAM FILLINGS
- MERCURY IN OTHER FORMS

- PESTICIDES AND HERBICIDES
- INSECTICIDES
- A DEATH IN THE FAMILY
- BROKEN HEART
- TAKING CARE OF A SICK LOVED ONE
- SPIDER BITE
- BEE STING
- ANTI-VIRAL PRESCRIPTION DRUGS
- OVERPRESCRIBED MEDICATIONS
- RECREATIONAL DRUG ABUSE
- FINANCIAL STRESS
- PHYSICAL INJURIES
- PROFESSIONAL CARPET CLEANING
- FRESH PAINT
- INSOMNIA
- TICK BITE- the red bulls eye is a sign that the tick is infected with borrelia.

ANTIBIOTICS

The conventional treatment of a Lyme diagnosis is with antibiotics because doctors think they are treating bacteria. This of course is a double-whammy to the immune system, since it kills off your good natural fighting bacterium. The virus, on the other hand, loves the antibiotics and feeds on it.

TESTING FOR LYME

You can have Lyme symptoms and receive negative test results since they are testing for the wrong thing...*Borrelia burgdorferi*

There are two primary tests:

- Enzyme-linked Immunosorbent Assay (ELISA)
- Western Blot

If you are having symptoms and test negative, chances are you have one of the many viruses causing the symptoms. Viral strains can also trigger false positives. The length of time to recover from your symptoms depends on your state of health, how long you've been ill and nutritional factors. The following recommendations, as well as Part IV, 'How to Finally Heal', will give you what you need to be free of Lyme symptoms.

HEALING FOODS

- Star Anise
- Asparagus
- Wild blueberries
- Radish
- Celery
- Cinnamon
- Garlic
- Apricot
- Onion

HEALING HERBS and SUPPLEMENTS

- Thyme
- Lemon balm
- Zinc
- Licorice root
- L-lysine
- Lomatium root
- Reishi mushrooms
- Silver Hydrosol
- Nascent iodine

PART IV

HOW TO FINALLY HEAL

CHAPTER XVII

Gut Health

The medical community has very little understanding of digestion, and may never fully understand the workings of the gut. Your gut is where your strength is, hence the expression, '*gut instinct*.' There is a definite emotion that controls good and bad bacteria in the gut. Poor gut health can hinder intuition.

UNDERSTANDING 'LEAKY-GUT'

Intestinal permeability has three sides:

1. *Conventional doctors-* leaky gut is a critical intestinal disease that perforates the lining of the intestines or stomach causing infections.
2. *Holistic doctors-* describes mold fungi like Candida, or bacteria creating holes in the walls of the intestines allowing toxins to leak into the blood stream.
3. *Williams' concept-* Ammonia permeability- when proteins reach the lower intestine completely undigested it lays there and rots. This putrefaction creates an ammonia gas that can cause bloating, digestive discomfort, chronic dehydration, or maybe no symptoms.

When good hydrochloric acid diminishes, bad acids take its place. This is the beginning of acid reflux and other such symptoms. Excess mucus can also develop at this point, with a lot of mucus coming up your throat for no apparent reason. The mucus can also travel down the intestinal tract and stop proper absorption of nutrients.

The theory discussed by William is that when food decomposes in the intestinal tract and produces ammonia, the toxic gas moves into the bloodstream creating havoc. Symptoms can include fatigue, skin problems, restless sleep, anxiety and the usual gut issues. It is not the Candida, therefore, expelling toxins through the intestinal walls as is commonly believed about leaky gut. (*See Conclusion for further comments.*)

Prescription drugs can disrupt the chemical balance of the gut, as can adrenaline. It interferes by slowly breaking down the digestive enzyme hydrochloric acid. You can rebuild hydrochloric acid by drinking daily, on an empty stomach, sixteen-ounces of fresh celery juice.

REMOVING TOXIC HEAVY METALS FROM THE GUT

Heavy metals are poisonous, especially if they oxidize, which creates cell damage. Their prime food is bad bacteria, virus, fungi and parasites. When the pathogens consume the heavy metals they release a neurotoxin gas that attaches itself to the ammonia gas and travels through the intestinal lining. This ultimately creates inflammation and many of the illnesses labeled as IBS, Crohn's, etc.

Options for removing heavy metals:

- Cilantro
- Parsley
- Zeolite
- Spirulina

- Garlic
- Sage
- L-glutamine
- Plantain leaf
- Red clover blossom

THE GUT'S NATURAL PROTECTION

William states that so far it has been undiscovered in medical research that we are born with tiny, furry hairs that line the intestinal tract. The hairs help to protect the gut from invasion of pathogens. It also sets up shop for the billions of good bacteria that keeps gut chemistry in balance.

PUBLISHER'S NOTE: *(We believe William is referring to villi, which was discovered and named decades ago.)*

To protect your villi, it is recommended to eat romaine, red leaf and butter lettuce, oregano, thyme, peppermint, bananas, apples, figs and dates. Stay away from the foods listed in Chapter XIX, "What Not to Eat".

RESTORING GUT FLORA and MAXIMIZING B12 PRODUCTION

Good bacteria in the gut produce B12, which is absorbed into the ileum. This is where methylation occurs. (He says science does not know this.) When methylation goes wrong:

- Bio-absorption of micronutrients is interrupted.
- Conversion process of vitamins and other nutrients is interrupted.
- A heightened level of homocysteine from a toxic liver or pathogens interferes with absorption of nutrients.

The ileum becomes inflamed when good bacteria throughout the gut is destroyed. When this occurs B12 plummets and the immune system is weakened. Use a B12 supplement (as methylcobalamin, blended with adenosylcobalamin) for easy conversion by the liver.

Rebuilding gut flora can be done with sprouted microorganisms such as:

- Alfalfa
- Broccoli
- Clover
- Fenugreek
- Lentil
- Mustard
- Sunflower
- Kale

Re-establishing hydrochloric acid, removing heavy metals, revising the ability to make B12 and restoring good bacteria, will heal gut problems.

GALLSTONES

To get rid of gallstones lower consumption of dense proteins and eat sodium-rich vegetables and fruits that contain healthy bio-acids. This includes spinach, kale, radishes, mustard greens, celery, lemons, oranges, grapefruit and limes.

Another method is to juice a handful of fresh, raw asparagus along with other juice ingredients.

FERMENTED FOODS

William states that the probiotics in fermented foods are not life-giving. They thrive off of the decay process. "They thrive off death, not life." The vast majority of fermented foods breed bacteria from foods that are no longer alive. They are foods of the past when there was little else to eat.

(See Conclusion for further comments.)

APPLE CIDER VINEGAR

ACV can be ideal for external use, such as addressing skin rashes, scalp issues, and even wounds. Any vinegar taken internally can be an irritant to the gut and ultimately detrimental.

PUBLISHER NOTE: *The acetic acid in ACV is very useful in balancing pH levels from acid to alkaline. Everything in the body works better in a neutral, to slightly alkaline environment and discourages the proliferation of all pathogens.*

CHAPTER XVIII

Freeing Your Brain and Body of Toxins

Toxic exposures to poisonous substances such as heavy metals, air pollution, pharmaceuticals, nanotechnology chemicals, pesticides, herbicides, fungicides, plastics, industrial cleaners, petroleum, dioxins, and thousands of others have seen a dramatic rise.

Most of us carry these toxins in our bodies our whole lives. Toxins pose multiple threats to your organs and immune system. They can also feed pathogens. Minimizing exposure and working on elimination is key to good health.

MERCURY

There was a time in the not too distant past when mercury was revered as a miraculous treatment doctors depended on. The use of mercury in the making of felt hats was also seen as harmless many years ago.

Fortunately, it was discovered that mercury is actually one of the most dangerous neurotoxins on the planet. Mercury absorbs into the cracks in our brain and fuels many diseases.

Mercury in the body has been accumulated through generations.

- **SEAFOOD**

Mercury is in all fish and contained in higher levels in tuna, swordfish, shark, and other large oily fish. You can mitigate the risk by eating small fish such as sardines and mackerel. Some wild salmon is also safe enough to eat in moderation.

- **DENTAL AMALGAMS**

Dental amalgam fillings are another source of mercury. Having them removed can be dangerous if not done properly. If the metal leaches into your system, it can lead to many types of illness. Remove only one at a time with a month in between. If you have had them removed it is time for cleanup. If new cavities occur, choose ceramic fillings instead.

***PUBLISHER'S NOTE**: Choose a biological dentist, when possible, who will use rubber dams and/or an oxygen mask when removing amalgam fillings. When a mercury filling is drilled it turns into vapor and can travel up the sinus passages crossing the blood/brain barrier.*

HEAVY METAL DETOX

Consuming the following five items daily will remove heavy metals.

- Barley grass juice extract powder; 1-2 tsp. mixed in water or juice.
- Spirulina (Hawaiian); 2 tsps. in water, coconut water, or juice.

- Cilantro; 1 cup in a smoothie, or juice, or add to salad or guacamole.
- Wild blueberries; eat at least 1 cup per day.
- Atlantic dulse; 2tbsp. of flakes daily, or same amount in strips.

Burdock root can be added to the protocol for an added boost. Chlorella has *unpredictability* and is less effective in *protection* from mercury.

WATER POLLUTION

Buy bottled water and be sure plastic containers are free of bisphenol. You can also purchase a high-quality water filter for your tap water. Be sure it filters heavy metals, chlorine, and fluoride. If you purchase a reverse-osmosis, or distillation system it removes all dissolved minerals also. You will have to buy ionic trace mineral drops to add back into your drinking water, since these are beneficial to your health.

Since the purification process deadens water, bring it back to life with a squeeze of lemon or lime.

- REMOVAL OF FLUORINE/CHLORINE

Blend equal parts blackberry leaf, raspberry leaf, hibiscus flower, and rose hips. Steep one tbsp. of the mixture per cup of hot water.

- PESTICIDES, HERBICIDES & FUNGICIDES

Most exposure is through conventional produce. Buy organic as much as possible and animal products that are free-range.

Parks and recreational areas are heavily sprayed with pesticides. Use a blanket to sit on the grass and wash afterwards.

Avoid spraying chemicals on your own lawn and try to refrain from insecticides in your home.

- REMOVAL OF PESTICIDES/ HERBICIDES/ FUNGICIDES

Blend equal parts burdock root, red clover, lemon verbena, and ginger. Steep one tbsp. of the mixture per cup of water.

- PLASTIC

There are plastics that cause inflammation, disrupt brain neurons, confuse hormones and feed cancers and pathogens. Use cloth bags as often as possible and glass containers to store food. Check for BPA-free and human-friendly plastics.

- PLASTIC REMOVAL

Blend equal parts fenugreek, mullein leaf, olive leaf, and lemon balm. Steep one tbsp. of the mixture per cup of hot water.

- CLEANERS

Industrial cleaners destroy dirt and germs, but are hazardous to humans also. Carpet cleaners are especially toxic. Opt for hard surfaces instead when you have a choice. There are many organic cleaners available now for all cleaning needs, including detergents. Dry cleaning especially, can be toxic and many dry cleaners have moved on to "green" cleaning. When you buy new clothes fabrics are usually coated in formaldehyde (which is cancer causing) so be sure to wash your new clothes before wearing.

- REMOVING CLEANING SOLVENTS

Blend calendula, chamomile, bladder wrack and borage in equal parts. Steep one tbsp. of the mixture per cup of hot water.

- RADIATION

Creatures higher up on the food chain absorb radiation from toxic exposures, and from incidents like Fukushima. Through bio-magnification the toxic matter accumulates in greater concentrations in creatures higher up the food chain.

Minimize dental x-rays. Be sure you are covered with a lead apron (including throat) when you do get dental x-rays. Do not automatically say yes to x-rays, only when necessary. For other medical procedures involving x-rays or radiation, be sure to weigh your options.

Sea vegetables can help to eliminate radiation by pulling it through the digestive tract. Select vegetables from the Atlantic, rather than the Pacific. They have a greater capacity to absorb toxins.

- REMOVING RADIATION

Blend Atlantic kelp, Atlantic dulse, dandelion leaf, and nettle leaf in equal parts. Steep one tbsp. of the mixture per cup of hot water.

MORE DETOX METHODS

- Lemon Water- drink 16 oz. of water with ½ a fresh lemon squeezed in it on waking. This helps to flush the toxins from the liver. You can also add a tsp. of raw honey and a tsp. of fresh grated ginger to the lemon water. It will help to restore glucose reserves to the liver and purge toxins.
- Aloe Vera Leaf Juice- fresh gel from the plant eaten daily can detox the liver and intestinal tract. The gel can be scooped from a filleted leaf and put into a smoothie or eaten directly.

- Juice Fasting- one-day fasting can be helpful. Choose celery, cucumbers, and apples. Be sure to juice 16-20 ounces every two-hours. The day should include six juices and at least 6 glasses of water. If you are bold you can add some spinach or kale and some ginger to taste. You can build up to a two-week fast to achieve impressive results.
- Water fasting- this is a more extreme detox and consists of a 16 oz. glass of water every hour. This gives your digestive system a vacation. Be sure to rest if necessary. You can try once per month for three months. Results can be amazing.
- Rebounding- a mini-trampoline ten-minutes per day creates circulation throughout the lymph system and encourages detoxification.
- Infrared Sauna- emits infrared light onto the skin for detox. Improves circulation, can remove toxins from the skin and help to eliminate aches and pains. Use for 15-20 minutes two times per week.
- Massage- promotes circulation to help with detox. Be sure to drink 16 oz. of lemon water after your massage to flush toxins.

CHAPTER XIX

What Not To Eat

FOODS HAZARDOUS TO YOUR HEALTH

CORN- most corn in the US is genetically modified (GMO). Corn and its by-products create inflammation and feeds pathogens. Try to avoid all corn and products that contain corn. This includes corn oils, high-fructose corn syrup, gluten-free products that substitute corn, and many other places where corn hides.

SOY- another crop that has been genetically modified. Many soy products also contain MSG. If you must eat soy stick to plain options, organic options or high-quality nama shoyu.

CANOLA OIL- another product the result of genetically modified plant. This oil creates inflammation, damaging to the digestive system, vascular damage, and a major cause of IBS. It has been touted as a health food, but is far from it. Avoid at all costs.

PROCESSED BEET SUGAR- another crop genetic modification. It feeds cancers, viruses, and bacteria. This is not the organic beet you eat raw, steamed or roasted. They are grown specifically to extract the sugar and are a hazard to your health.

EGGS- William states that eggs can be a tremendous support for those with Lyme, Lupus, Chronic fatigue, etc., but a prime food for cancer, cysts and other growths. Eggs can cause inflammation and allergies and trigger edema.

DAIRY- contains fat, which is difficult for the digestive system and liver to process. The combination of lactose, fat and sugar has a negative effect on health. It is mucus producing and can contain hormones, antibiotics, soy and corn.

PORK- avoid all pork products, including ham and bacon. This is due to its high fat content.

FARMED FISH- many times fish bread in small areas have parasites, collect algae and other issues. They are then given antibiotics and the water can also be treated with chemicals. Choose wild fish instead, such as salmon, haddock or halibut.

GLUTEN- grains contain protein called gluten that can be very difficult to digest. This includes wheat, barley, rye, and spelt. Even oats can become contaminated with the gluten protein. They are all contaminated with multiple allergens and cause inflammation, bloating, and other symptoms. Gluten can trigger Crohn's, colitis and other disorders. *(**PUBLISHER'S NOTE**: It is also responsible for celiac disease.)*

MSG- monosodium glutamate is a food additive that causes numerous allergic reactions for many. It is especially harmful if you have an illness affecting your brain or central nervous system. It is essential to read labels, since it is included in thousands of products as a flavor enhancer. If you see these names on a label, you know there is MSG in the product:

Glutamate, hydrolyzed, autolyzed, protease, carrageenan, maltodextrin, sodium caseinate, balsamic vinegar, barley malt, malt extract, yeast extract, brewer's yeast, corn starch, wheat start, modified food starch, gelatin, textured protein, whey protein, soy protein, soy sauce, broth, bouillon, stock, and seasoning.

NATURAL FLAVORS- definitely code for 'MSG.' Unfortunately the FDA approved this labeling!

ARTIFICIAL FLAVORS- as they are rightfully named, artificial, meaning chemical compounds.

ARTIFICIAL SWEETENERS- most contains aspartame, a neurotoxin. They are disruptive to neurons and the central nervous system. Can cause strokes in the brain. Eating fruit is a better choice.

CITRIC ACID- not as bad as other additives. It is usually corn derived and not the same as naturally occurring citric acid in the body. It can cause stomach distress.

SUPPLEMENTS TO AVOID

L-CARNITINE- feeds herpes viruses. Stay away especially in a concentrated form.

GLANDULAR SUPPLEMENTS- made from bovine or other animal sources are prime foods for cancers, virus and bacteria.

WHEY PROTEIN- creates inflammation and may include MSG.

FISH OIL SUPPLEMENTS- since fish contains mercury, and other dioxins, it is not possible to remove them. Stay away from all of these supplements. Instead look for plant-based, algae derived omega supplements.

IRON SUPPLEMENTS- iron feeds on viruses and most with anemia have an underlying virus. Choose plant-based iron products.

CHAPTER XX

Fruit Fear

In recent years, Americans have lowered their fruit consumption by as much as 15%. There has been a widespread cry across health platforms, conventional and otherwise, to lower, or cut out fruit consumption due to its sugar content. Low-carb diets have been the craze!

Without fruit, fertility is at risk. Fertility depends on the fructose and glucose that occurs in fruit, as well as the phytochemicals bonded to the sugars. Fruit has many other essential ingredients important to fertility.

Humans have cultivated fruit for thousands of years. Scurvy is a disease due to a Vitamin C deficiency. In years past, it was the lower class, which did not have access to fruit, which held the highest rate of scurvy.

William states that seasonal eating is over-rated and it is a crime to not be eating the foods that are shipped to us from other regions. You are robbing yourself of disease-protecting nutrients. Limiting fruit in your diet will increase your chances of illness and shorten your life expectancy.

There is also no issue with picking un-ripe fruit (except for berries). It still ripens to its full nutritional level after being picked. Also, grafting and hybridization, or crossbreeding, is not an issue. These are safe techniques to create new varieties of fruit.

Fruit has properties that soothe the adrenal glands, strengthen the endocrine system, repair, revitalize and restore other functions and systems in the body. Glucose is the number one fuel in the body and glucose is derived from the sugar in fruit. The body craves glucose and when you cut out fruit you will eat other foods, not as healthy, to feed that craving.

Fruit is best eaten by itself, or when paired with raw vegetables, especially leafy greens. They are both digested quickly, in contrast to protein, fats, and complex carbohydrates. Eat those foods about an hour *after* you eat your fruit.

Fruit is anti-cancerous and fights cancer more effectively than any other food. (Its also heavily sprayed and the pesticides seep into the fruit. Only tough skinned- fruit is clean. Cancer cannot feed off of the sugar in fruit and instead delivers the benefits of the antioxidants and other nutrients attached to the sugars. Fruit also kills virus and bacteria. The most powerful are bananas, wild blueberries, apples and papayas.

The sugar in fruit does not feed Candida, since it is broken down within minutes in the stomach and goes into the bloodstream. As a result, it never reaches the Candida in the intestinal tract.

PUBLISHERS NOTE: *There would be no blood circulation for this to be true.*

Fruit sugar does not hinder the liver. Fruit protects the liver by giving it the store of glucose it needs to function properly. Fruit is your friend...it does not cause illness. No other food is as effective at preventing disease, killing pathogens, and repairing the body. Fruit prevents oxidation, which is the process that ages us.

Wild blueberries are at the top of the list as a powerful brain food, the most anti-oxidant rich food, and can prevent and reverse disease.

CHAPTER XXI

The 28-Day Healing Cleanse

THE PLAN

For four weeks, eat only raw fruits and vegetables. If your health is in dire straits, or if you have a lot of weight to loose, this time frame can be extended. If this is not possible, even one week is likely to bring results.

OR:

Choose one cleanse day per week.

William says this plan works because it maximizes the nutrition you get in every meal. The uncooked fruits and vegetables are digested quickly and easily. The body will re-mineralize, alkalize, detoxify and mend. The living food, full of enzymes, will bring you back to life. Limit your salt intake and hydrate with plenty of water, coconut water, herbal tea and fresh fruit juice.

If you have a specific diagnosis that is listed previously in the book, add those foods and supplements also to the protocol.

EARLY MORNING

Start every day with a cleansing beverage. That could be lemon water, cucumber juice, celery juice, coconut water, an herbal tea or any other choices previously listed. Water is ok… just being sure to drink.

BREAKFAST

Fruit smoothie; combine fruits of your choice with added greens. (Fruit being the main component.)

MID-MORNING

Another fruit smoothie, either what you made earlier, or a new blend.

LUNCH

Make a salad of mixed greens, maybe cabbage and sprouts; add in fruits of your choice. Dressing can be a blended avocado, some cilantro and juice of two oranges.

MID-AFTERNOON

Snack on fruits of your choice, possibly celery sticks and some raw honey.

DINNER

Make a creamy spinach soup in the blender. Add tomatoes, celery stalk, juice of an orange, cilantro and a clove of garlic. Can be poured over veggies noodles, like cucumber. If there are digestion issues stay away from raw zucchini.

EVENING

Snack on an apple and a date.

MODIFICATIONS

Switch up your ingredients daily. You can even switch the lunch and dinner. The decision is yours to repeat the same meals, or keep changing. You can change up the dressing by topping off the salad with guacamole and limejuice.

If you have blood sugar issues, keep grazing all day. A super power cleanse is by cutting out the avocado so there is no fat in the diet and eliminate any extra salt.

If you prefer a less intense cleanse you can steam or roast your vegetables with coconut oil; or make a soup with mixed vegetables. You can also use this method to transition in or out of the raw diet.

You may become emotional and need extra support, or need more rest during the cleanse. For spiritual support turn to the next two chapters.

TRANSITIONING

When you come to the end of the cleanse, do not jump back into your usual diet. Gradually work your way back in so as not to overload your digestive system. You decide how long to stay on the diet, which can be continued for an extended period by adding some fats or a cooked meal here or there. Some need more protein than others and your body will let you know what it needs.

Consult 'Conclusion' for additional suggestions.

CHAPTER XXII

Soul-Healing Meditations and Techniques

Everyone is soul-searching. It takes different forms for different people. Everyone deserves to be healthy and happy. William says the following are the secrets to reviving your soul and spirit, finding peace, and feeling whole again.

EMOTIONAL DETOX

When going through a physical detox, you may experience an emotional detox. Emotions can bubble up as toxins leave the body. This is a temporary phase. Your goal is to release negative emotions and move forward. Meditation can help you to let go, claim your life that God wants you to.

FORMS OF MEDITATION

William says, "Meditation is a state of being that rewires your subconscious to be more at peace, which heals your soul."

Meditation can take many forms...bike riding, a walk in the park, music, dancing, etc. Whatever makes you feel positive and hopeful will bring healing to your body and soul.

The following are some methods of meditation taught by Spirit...

WAVES ON THE BEACH

Envision every wave, while sitting, standing or walking, as a surge of soul-cleansing energy. As a wave comes in, imagine it scrubbing away old wounds and scrubbing loose damaging emotions. As the wave recedes, watch it take away the impurities. With each new wave be cleansed of poisonous memories and see them wash out to sea. Wading in the water also brings the energy to you to envision the things you want in your life.

You can also call upon the Angel of the Ocean, which you'll learn more about in the next chapter.

SURROUNDED BY TREES

To bring in the gifts of nature call upon the Angel of the Trees. Acknowledge the peaceful environment and turn your attention to their root system. Think about their process of pulling water and minerals from the earth. Imagine roots growing from your feet and into the energy of mother earth. When you feel at peace and complete, breakaway knowing your roots are there for you to draw healing energy from whenever needed.

This powerful grounding exercise will help you to free yourself from fear and to strengthen body and soul.

FREE AS A BIRD

Birdsongs are sacred music. Their frequencies resonate deep within us and can heal disease. Observing birds can be powerful and ignites and unleashes the spirit. Activate healing by watching the actions of birds in flight and how they land with a sense of safety and bring that into your own soul.

Hummingbirds are light-workers. When you spot one recognize they are a symbol of light. They are like a fairy, spreading the light of the angels. Let it purify your thoughts and send them off with your wish to be carried to where it needs to go.

BEE WATCHING

Step into a meditation as you watch a bee fly from flower to flower, pollinating as he goes. Their frequency can heal disease and promote soul restoration. Tell your cells to vibrate at the frequency of the bee and to resonate with their healing vibration.

COLLECTING STONES

To remove negative emotions, take a walk in nature. Look for three stones that resonate with you. Name each one by the emotion you harbor. Develop a relationship with them by keeping them on your nightstand. The healing frequencies of the minerals will help to release the emotions. When you feel healed from them, bring the stones back to nature and release them into water. The water will purify them and you'll both be purified.

SUNBATHING

To derive benefit from the sun, spend time each day letting your skin absorb its' warmth. Acclimate to fifteen minutes per day. If it is winter, sit by a sun-filled window. Call upon the Angel of the Sun to help your soul take in the rays to heal your body.

PICKING FRUIT

Meditate on the abundance from nature that is brought to us in fruit. It is living food attached to the plant. Fruit picking can be a unique form of healing as we appreciate the bounties of the earth. Take the time to focus on the rhythm of its' growth, from seed to plant, to flower to fruit. Our own lives go through a similar development. Taking in and focusing on the trust and faith within will bring about a fruitful life.

WATCHING YOUR GARDEN GROW

Gardening is an opportunity to absorb the sounds of nature, which are healing. Weeding can be turned into a meditation by imagining each weed you pull as an ill thought or negative emotion to be removed. Make room for abundance in your life. Even in an apartment you can have pots on your windowsill or balcony.

EXERCISING CREATIVITY

Create art and attract an audience from the angelic realm. Angels witness every time we are creative. You will gain new meaning with an understanding that the Angels of creativity are watching. Whenever you are creating something, even packing lunch, imagine the angels cheering you on and making an imprint in the heavens.

RESTORING TRUST WITH SUNSETS

Emotional blows can create soul damage. They also hinder your ability to believe you can overcome illness. To heal this become aware of sunsets. At the end of the day take a few moments to watch the sunset (not looking directly into the sun.)

You may feel a sense of loss as the darkness takes over. Call in the Angel of Trust and embrace the knowledge and trust that the sun will rise tomorrow. Do this at least three times per week to change your perspective on life.

The next morning, on rising, bask in the idea that the sun has returned and will never let you down and your soul will relearn trust. This will activate healing energy.

GAZING BEYOND THE STARS

God keeps an essence of our souls in case we lose ourselves. It is not uncommon for a soul to become damaged, which is why this safety mechanism exists.

To reclaim your soul, spend a little time each evening gazing up into the sky. Connect with the stars, and then focus on the space beyond the stars. Remind yourself that part of you resides there, unharmed. By repeating this exercise for just a few minutes each time your soul regenerates.

WHO DO YOU WORK FOR?

You work for GOD! Repeat this exercise every day to yourself and your perspective will change. When this happens the result will change how you feel and interact with everyone around you. Your purpose will shine through. If you feel overwhelmed, connecting with this phrase will help you to find new ways of approaching the work.

PUBLISHER'S NOTE: *You may have success with the author's 'Meditations', if you are looking for something more read the Conclusion for instructions to the first step to the gateway to the subconscious; reaching ALPHA. Only by attaining this control can you drop into a healing state.*

CHAPTER XXIII

Essential Angels

Everyone has the right and ability to reach out to angels whenever needed. Angels have always been with us to help us adapt and survive. We are never alone. When we arrive there is a certain role for us, the angels help us to fulfill that role, if we choose. The angels are here to guide us, help us grow, bring opportunities, pull us out of darkness, and show us the light. They are not here to grant our every wish; they help us to do God's work.

You have to know the right angels to ask and the right way to ask. You have to be open, have faith and work with them.

Archangel Michael and Archangel Gabriel are the two most well known angels. They are very popular, have free will and choose who and where they work. We will talk about other Angels you can call upon. They are female and known by a word of power.

THE TWENTY-ONE ESSENTIAL ANGELS

The number twenty-one stands for rebirth, new beginnings, reclamation, and fresh starts. These are the ones most powerful and beneficial in today's times. Each is potent and has different properties. You can call upon them individually or as a team.

- **ANGEL OF MERCY**- by far the most powerful to call upon in times of darkness.
- **ANGEL OF FAITH**- call upon her daily to turn into a habit. Tell the Angel you are ready.
- **ANGEL OF TRUST**- for struggling with betrayal
- **ANGEL OF HEALING**- for temporary relief, or to heal a loved one. For long-term healing other Angels are needed.
- **ANGEL OF RESTITUTION**- to help recover from emotional trauma and resolve deep-seated issues.
- **ANGEL OF DELIVERANCE**- dealing with earthly judgment; can help free the soul from fear, anger, or deception.
- **ANGEL OF SUN**- when you are in the sun call for her to open cells to the healing power of the rays.
- **ANGEL OF LIGHT**- more powerful than the light on earth, or that from the sun, name her to be bathed in restorative light.
- **ANGEL OF WATER**- ask that the frequency of the water you bathe in be more cleansing, nourishing, and grounding. When soaking a wound, ask her to quicken the healing.
- **ANGEL OF AIR**- to cleanse negative vibrations from the air after negative encounters. This can also help to change your frame of mind.
- **ANGEL OF PURITY**- to break free from addictions
- **ANGEL OF FERTILITY**- for aid in conception and carrying to term.

- **ANGEL OF BIRTH**- for health of mother and baby during delivery.
- **ANGEL OF PEACE**- to help heal mental distress and bring in hope and positivity.
- **ANGEL OF BEAUTY**- when you are cut off from nature and need to bring in its beauty; to help shift people's mindset off of physical beauty and to recognize the beauty of the soul.
- **ANGEL OF PURPOSE**- when you are confused or worried about your purpose and losing confidence call on the Angel.
- **ANGEL OF KNOWLEDGE**- when need information or advice, or would like to help another, call on this Angel for guidance.
- **ANGEL OF WISDOM**- for guidance with important decisions
- **ANGEL OF AWARENESS**- to help to be mindful and more in the moment; also for those around you to be better communicators and less judgmental.
- **ANGEL OF RELATIONSHIPS**- to attract a relationship, or to improve one.
- **ANGEL OF DREAMS**- call upon her to help re-experience soul freedom and/or to enter your dreams to help sort out issues.

UNKNOWN ANGELS

There are 144,000 unknown Angels who do not have names. They have no ego, since they have no notoriety. They are the most powerful and least in demand. They can perform miracles, if you have faith in them. You might call upon the Angel of Light during waking hours to restore your soul, and then at night call upon the Unknown Angels to help with chronic illness while asleep. You can ask for one, or a group to help you.

ACCESSING ANGELS

You have to ask for help out-loud! You can't just *think* it. Angels have free will and do not want to be stuck in everyone's thoughts. Speaking your desires shows them you are sincere and committed. Using this method is like making a phone call and ordering a delivery. It is a process of will and intention. Be sure to focus your attention and be willing to receive her.

If you are deaf, or have speech impairment, use sign language or ask the Angel of deliverance to carry your soul's wishes.

You can talk to the Angels about specific out comes, but do not be surprised if it is not what you expected. What you receive may not be an outcome you even anticipated.

If you start tapping into the power of the Angels you get to move forward in your life, to heal, and to have good things happen.

AFTERWORD

Keep the Faith

Most people on earth today lose faith, even if they believe in God. Part of the reason things go wrong is because there is a loss of faith. A lack of believing in good in the world causes negative consequences. When we lose faith, a sense of higher purpose follows. This is how industries end up dumping toxic substances that cause illness, as well as many other inherently bad decisions that occur.

So many are ill today and disheartened by a world of disappointment and fear. Always come back to the truth, "*You are allowed to live a good life. You deserve to live a good life. A good life exists in you. And the foundation of a good life is good health. You deserve to heal, to tap into your body's restorative mechanisms. You deserve to be happy and well.*"

Don't lose touch with your essence and conviction only to make bad decisions. Faith is your most powerful tool. Here is a visualization to access your faith:

1. Envision *faith* as a golden rope, a lifeline trailing from the sky
2. Grasp the rope, pulling on it like ringing a bell in the heavens

Overtime faith will trickle down to you; enter your heart, soul, spirit, and body. You will restore yourself to health as your faith begins to build. It takes practice and patience.

Your life can transform as you take the lessons in this book to heart.

> *"God, Spirit, and the Angelic Realm really want us to thrive. Just as one candle can pass its flame to thousands more, you'll be the light in the world that can ignite the faith of countless others."*

PUBLISHER'S CONCLUSION

Health care and healing falls into three categories:

- Conventional Mainstream Medicine
- Natural based, Holistic, Alternative, Integrative medicine
- Everything else

The first two listed are self-explanatory. The third encompasses the category of faith healing, energy modalities and the like. This book falls under the third category. Since William states he has no medical training and the information is brought to him from a third-party source, it would therefore, be faith and trust that would entice one to follow the protocols.

Having said that, it is always a good idea, when embarking on a change in diet, or adding a new regimen of supplements and herbs to do your homework. As an example, if you have disturbed digestion, you may not be able to embark on a diet of *raw* foods for any length of time. First try it for a day, or ease into it by alternating steamed or roasted vegetables with a raw meal. Be diligently aware of your symptom picture as you make the changes. If it is not a fit, stop.

By the same token, you may not do well abruptly eliminating *meat* from your diet. Possibly ease into this change with protein once per day initially, then once every other day, then once in the week. Chances are if your body allows, you can now take the leap.

Easing in and out of the 28-Day healing cleanse described in Chapter XXI, or any dramatic dietary change, can be the key to success. The following is a vegetable soup recipe from Dr. Bieler. Henry G. Bieler (April 2, 1893 – October 11, 1975) was an American physician, best known for his book "Food is Your Best Medicine." Bieler was the famous doctor to the stars in the 50's and 60's who healed with food, rather than a prescription pad. His treatments proved that removing toxicity from the body cures most illness. The secret to this amazing soup is that it can efficiently flush the liver and kidneys, while helping to restore gut balance. The following is his original recipe:

Bieler's Soup

1 lb. Cut Green Beans

2-3 Celery Stalks (if your digestion can tolerate)

4-6 Zucchini, thickly sliced

Handful of fresh Parsley

Buy Organic…

Place all the ingredients in a pot, cover with water, bring to a boil, and simmer for a few more minutes until beans are tender. Remove from the heat and let sit uncovered for 5 minutes. Pour into a blender and mix well.

This can be eaten thick in a bowl as soup, or thinned as a drink. Use more or less water, according to your taste. Can be served hot or cold. This soup can substitute for any meal or as a between meal snack. It becomes a powerful detox when you incorporate it three times per day, for a period of time.

SUPPLEMENTS

Supplements are another important area that needs investigation and *discernment.* Taking handfuls of supplements daily can be as detrimental to some as taking none at all. If you have poor digestion you will only be able to breakdown and metabolize the supplements appropriate to your particular situation.

The supplements and herbs listed in the text after each illness are easily searchable online. There are no unusual or unique ingredients revealed in the text. Check out their use, why you would need them, and which might be redundant.

As an example, Chapter XV discusses William's concept of lowered hormones at menopause having health advantages. The list of supplements that follows includes supplements that are known to raise hormone levels.

Another inconsistency shows up throughout the book regarding fats. That fats are bad, carbs are good. Yet many of the lists of healing supplements include adding back into your diet EPA & DHA omega fats. He discusses using plant sources of omega fats, since fish based omegas are contaminated with heavy metals. This is certainly true for some brands however the process of *distillation* removes metals. With a little research you can find such brands.

Perhaps you need hydrochloric acid, as discussed in a previous chapter. If so, be sure this is appropriate for you. As an example, before attempting a protocol for HCL, it would be wise to do an acid test to determine if this is an issue for you. Try this method...the next time you have heartburn take a tablespoon of apple cider vinegar (ACV). If it alleviates the heartburn, then you are in need of HCL. If it however aggravates, this means you are too acidic and should avoid HCL, as well as all vinegars.

Speaking of being too acidic, this is a topic not covered in this text. Possibly William felt it was not necessary because the recommended diet, for the most part, is an alkaline diet. However, knowing why you need to do something is always a compelling reason to stick to it. For example, some fruit can be very acidic (oranges) and you would not want to unknowingly be choosing acidic fruits regularly.

There is no virus, or other pathogen that can survive long-term in an alkaline environment. What does this mean? It means it is imperative to regularly monitor your pH.

The human body is comprised of approximately 70% water. To be healthy all that water needs to have a healthy pH balance, not too acid, not too alkaline. The letters "pH" mean "potential of hydrogen" and simply measure how acid or alkaline the body is on a scale of 0-14. Optimum health is achieved when the body stays in a slightly alkaline environment at about 7.0-7.5, as measured by saliva.

Many drugstores carry pH strips to test saliva, or they can be purchased online. Anyone experiencing acid-reflux, or other digestive symptoms will test below the neutral level of 7.0 which means digestion cannot function properly in this acidic state.

An alkaline diet that restores a healthy pH balance goes a long way to improving many symptoms. The added bonus is that pathogens, like a virus, die off! It is through an alkaline environment that you will have an easier time ridding the body of toxins and pathogens.

Bottom line...before you make a decision to change your diet or supplement protocols, investigate and choose wisely so that you have the very best results possible. Keep in mind that what works for one person does not necessarily work for another. Also, don't hesitate to seek the opinion of a trained professional. The money you spend for a consultation with a qualified practitioner far outweighs bad choices that may ultimately adversely impact your health.

To complete this summary, let's look at:

WHAT WE KNOW & WHAT WE DON'T KNOW...

INTRODUCTION

William says he reveals health ideas and concepts not known to the medical community as yet. Through our research, this is not exactly correct. Ideas and concepts discussed throughout exist either within conventional medical literature, or within a number of different branches of natural, holistic, alternative integrative medical writings and practices that William may not be aware of? Some other concepts introduced seem contrary to basic science, biology, or logic.

Having said that, as I mentioned previously, this book is not meant to trash or demean the work of Anthony William. It is instead a summary of the work, with questions, additions and corrections where appropriate. William is sincere in revealing that he has no formal training in the topics he covers.

CHAPTER I ORIGINS OF THE MEDICAL MEDIUM

The Spirit tells William that only one or two people per century are given the gift of communication. Most are familiar with Edgar Cayce (1877-1945) who 'channeled' health, as well as other predictions for his followers. Padre Pio (1887 – 1968), was another mystic who shared messages from another source. They are two in recorded history, from the last century, who were well documented.

William further states that he is unique from other mediums because he can ask Spirit at any time and any place for instant information. We do not know if Cayce or Pio possessed this ability? Since we are lacking historical documentation in this area it remains unknown at this time.

CHAPTER III EBV, CHRONIC FATIGUE & FIBROMYALGIA

In regards to the statement William makes that the medical community is aware of only one strain of Epstein-Barr virus, this is not accurate. The following is from the government website, PubMed.

> *"The publication of EBV genome 1984 led to several studies regarding the identification of different viral strains. Currently, EBV is divided into EBV type 1 (B95-8 strain) and EBV type 2 (AG876 strain), also known as type A and type B, which have been distinguished based upon genetic differences in the Epstein-Barr nuclear antigens (EBNAs) sequence. Several other EBV strains have been described in the past 10 years considering variations on EBV genome."*

William further states that traditionally, doctors have had no treatment for EBV, until he brought to light the answers. This statement may be true among the conventional medical community in America however; there are numerous successful treatments for EBV and other virus within other branches of medicine, such as Chinese, Ayerveda, and in European medical systems with the use of Homeopathy, as well as Pleomorphic Medicine. The real issue probably lays in missed and undiagnosed cases of the viruses.

CHAPTER VI DIABETES & HYPOGLYCEMIA

Regarding thyroid medications, William states correctly that thyroid medicine does not go after the root cause of thyroid disorder. He further states that they instead add hormones to the blood stream in the hopes the body will use them to replace the hormones the thyroid is not producing. The correction is that the thyroid *regulates* hormones it does not *produce* hormones.

CHAPTER IX CANDIDA

William does not believe it to be true that Candida cuts through the lining of the intestines and causes leaky gut.

Candida is a natural part of the digestive system, but when it overgrows it does get through the mucus lining. When this happens there is no protection from virus and bacteria going into the blood stream. They are no longer trapped in the intestines.

William states that a high-fat, high-protein diet does not starve Candida, but instead feeds it. What we do know is that Candida is a *fungus and fungus feeds on sugars*, not protein or good fats.

CHAPTER X MIGRAINES

Migraines are the result of sluggish lymph fluid. A Migraine is like a short circuit, which is why there is sensitivity to light. Lymph fluid is water and that water needs flushing and cleansing.

CHAPTER XI SHINGLES

William states that, contrary to medical science, chicken pox has no connection to the Shingles virus. What we do know is that the science-based evidence tells us the opposite, since they are in fact derived from the same virus. (Unless our microscopes are missing something?)

CHAPTER XII ADHD & AUTISM

"Mercury can be transmitted from the mother while in the womb and from fathers at conception." Mercury can definitely pass from mother to baby; however, since sperm is known to be *pure* heavy metal contamination cannot be passed from the father during conception.

In the discussion regarding heavy metal detox he says the situation created by heavy metals sets up by age four and can be removed if dealt with before the age of eighteen. By this age, the midline of the brain *closes* limiting the free-flow of energy. We do know that the mid-line *never* closes, or there would be no communication between the left and right sides of the brain.

In discussing dietary choices for detoxification William stresses a low fat, low protein, high carbohydrate diet since the brain runs on sugars. We do know that the brain is made up of 70% fat; therefore, it is not sugars or glucose that supports this structure.

Glucose is a fast burning fuel, a fight or flight chemical, not designed to run the brain, just helps us to get out of the way. Medium chain triglycerides (MCT oil) pass the blood brain barrier and is the fuel that runs the brain. It is the insulator. The brain is a transformer and needs fat to insulate the brain so it does not short circuit. Glucose gives a sugar rush and too much of it can short-circuit the brain. Sugar is a fat-burning carbon in the brain. Fat is there to move the body, *not sugar*.

Tantamount to this conversation is the clarification between good fats and bad fats. They are:

- **Trans fats/ Saturated fats** - partially hydrogenated vegetable oils (Bad)
- **Unsaturated fats**- animal products, (OK in moderation)

- **Polyunsaturated fats-** essential oils, omega-3, fish (Good)
- **Monosaturated fats-** nuts, avocado, olive oil (Good)

CHAPTER XV PREMENSTRUAL SYNDROME AND MENOPAUSE

There was a time, not so long ago, when women NEVER discussed their female issues, even to each other. There has been a long recorded history of shame, embarrassment and humiliation brought on by men regarding this topic. Even today in countries like India and Africa women are shunned by the life-giving cycle of a woman. The idea that PMS and menopausal symptoms did not exist prior to the 1950's is merely another example of the ignorance of men. Most of what is written in this chapter falls under this category.

CHAPTER XVII GUT HEALTH

FERMENTATION

William discusses the idea that fermented foods are NOT life-giving and should not be eaten.

Actually, when cabbage *ferments* it breaks down into the perfect balance of enzymes manufactured in the pancreas. Also, fermentation is a process of *live* food. If it were dead, it would not be fermenting. It is creating natural hydrochloric acid. As far as the statements regarding fermentation yielding bacteria...yes, of course, good bacteria that is the foundation of gut chemistry.

The best fertilizers are those made from fermented foods, since they supply pre-digested nutrients to proliferate the life of the plants. It is called composting.

APPLE CIDER VINEGAR

We commented on this topic in the chapter itself regarding Williams' concept that fermented food is bad for you. Here we have added another comment.

The maltic acid in ACV helps to prevent gallstones & kidney stones by breaking up the amalgamation of calcium. The potassium & sodium are the proper ratio for healthy blood pressure. This is well documented in the 1953 Nobel Prize for Medicine in the discovery of the citric-acid cycle.

CHAPTER XVIII FREEING YOUR BRAIN AND BODY OF TOXINS

William mentions that chlorella is trendy and 'unpredictable', therefore does not recommend its use. He is probably referring to brands derived from unclean sources. If you can access a verifiable organic source, chlorella is one of the most powerful heavy metal detoxification ingredients known.

William further states, "Chlorella is *irresponsible* when it comes down to protecting you from the hazards of mercury." Protecting you from mercury is not the function of chlorella. Since it is capable of efficiently crossing the blood/brain barrier it is a powerful tool in pulling the mercury, and other metals from the cells. But don't stop there; once the metals are mobilized they need to be flushed. Cilantro is a good choice to help complete this task.

CHAPTER XIX WHAT NOT TO EAT

The food list contained in this chapter rightfully points out the dangers of genetically modified foods (GMO). GMO foods are well documented as being inflammatory and an irritant to the immune system.

Eggs is in a different category. There are some who are allergic to eggs and this is usually due to their sensitivity to Sulphur. For millions of others eggs are a staple food, especially if you cannot tolerate gluten, dairy, soy, or other food categories.

Under 'Supplements' William lists Glandulars as a category to stay away from. In Europe this system of medicine is referred to as '*Organotherapy*'. There is much written on the topic. It has been used safely and effectively for decades by many well-known medical doctors. The sources of supply are clean, highly regulated and has brought many back from the brink of chronic illness. Standard Process is probably the most well-known brand of supplements in America that successfully include glandulars in their formulas.

CHAPTER XXII SOUL HEALING MEDITATIONS

If a meditation practice is of interest to you the following will further your success.

Here is a simple meditation gifted from a Master.

The Gateway to the Subconscious...

There are five levels of brainwaves, *Gamma, Beta, Alpha, Theta and Delta. Beta* is our waking state and *Alpha* is the resting state of the brain. It is access to *Alpha* that is necessary to reach a meditative state.

The mental force of *healing* is the ability to enter into the *Alpha state.* There can be no healing until you turn off the thinking side of your brain. This is why sleep is crucial to healing, since we heal while we sleep. When we turn off stress hormones the healing process can begin. The peace you find in the following meditation is the same peace you feel on drifting off to sleep.

Very few have an understanding of how to get to Alpha quickly and easily. Here is the secret:

COUNTING DOWN TO ALPHA

Learn to invoke pattern recognition and the brain turns itself off. This method must be spoken *IN YOUR HEAD* to be effective. You will count down from three to zero. Each number is repeated twice and by the time you reach zero you will have reached the relaxed state of Alpha.

SCREAM...in your head (You may have to practice this initially.)

Scream 3	PAUSE	QUIETER	3	PAUSE	QUIETER still
2	PAUSE	QUIETER	2	PAUSE	QUIETER (WHISPER)
1	PAUSE	QUIETER	1	PAUSE	QUIETER
0	PAUSE	IF NECESSARY 0...			

If you do this exercise every day for two weeks you will no longer have the need to count down. Merely the *intent* will bring you to Alpha.

The following is a simple, but effective Pre-Meditation (Prayer) to ground you prior to any meditation you choose.

I am more than my body...

I am more than my circumstances...

I am here and nowhere else...

I am as the Creator made me

And I have the DNA of God running through my veins.

I am you, and you are me.

That is who I am.

When you state who you are and why you are here, it sets up a sense of purpose.

CHAPTER XXIII ESSENTIAL ANGELS

Hard to know exactly how to comment on this final chapter, except to say that the reader can do their own due-diligence and research the status and disposition of Angels in Scripture. We will say...

- Angels do not have human attributes...*free will* is a *human* attribute.
- All things in existence are *named*, if they are not named, they do not exist. This is a law of Divine Providence.

We hope you have enjoyed this summary and analysis with the inclusion of corrections and additions, where appropriate. It is our sincere hope that whatever decisions you make in your health choices and spiritual teachings they bring you to a heightened state of health, happiness, and peace.

Made in the USA
Middletown, DE
23 July 2022

69934628R00066